'The average person spends 140 hours per week not moving, that only leaves 28 hours of motion. This includes walking to and from the house to the car, from the car to the office and then from the office to the car. The demands put on our bodies have drastically changed...for the worse'

DESCRIPTION OF TERMS

I have kept most of the book fairly straightforward but here are a few terms you may not know…YET.

-*Myofascial Meridians*-

Myo(muscle)Fascia(connective tissue)

-*Foundational*-

Refers to movement patterns that we are born to do. As infants we learn the basic crawling, sitting, kneeling, rolling and then progress to standing, walking, running, climbing, jumping. Bending, twisting and reaching come as we develop more task oriented.

-*Adapted*-

This refers to more specific patterns used in sport or in adding resistance to sitting creates the squat or to bending creates deadlifts.

-*Lymphatic System*-

It's the only system that requires movement to function. It transports healthy white blood cells and disposes of toxins throughout the entire body.

PREFACE

The ability to move pain free eludes most of us on a daily basis, as we carry on throughout each day doing the same things over and over we have learned to live with discomfort. And what may start as aches here and there will turn into chronic pain over time. The demands that our bodies are under have changed dramatically since our given design and evolution. The need to walk long distance, climb, crawl and run both from predators and towards our prey has given way to sitting in the same position at work, while driving and even when spending time with family around the table or watching our favourite shows.

The foundation hasn't changed, only how we use and treat or in many cases, how we mistreat our bodies. Many of my clients have reached a last-ditch-effort feeling and because the majority of modalities of therapy are Band-Aids only, the pain comes back and it is often worse. I am not saying that other methods are not helpful, rather I am pointing out that the only real fix is change. If you suffer from back pain due to a certain fascial posture you have adapted then nothing will correct it outside of changing the pattern or position.

Moving is the cure for all that ails you. Move more and move often.

INTRODUCTION

Welcome to a guidebook that is designed to help you discover a body that can function without pain. The movements in this guidebook are designed to help the 9-5 office workers. They are simple to learn and only require your full commitment. Doing them once in a while will give you exactly that, temporary relief. However, implementing them into your weekly schedule will not only get you moving, it will change how your body feels day-to-day.

I spent Thirty-five years of my life playing sports, training like an athlete and believe me my body paid the price. I could never have imagined that at Forty, I would feel better both mentally and physically than when I was thirty. Everyone says that at forty your body will ache but it doesn't have to. What must change is your perception of fitness and how to do it correctly. One of the biggest obstacles my clients face when they come see me, is letting go of the notion that high intensity training is some how helping them counteract sitting all day. It simply is not true and honestly it is making tension worse.

So does that mean you can't go have a hard workout, of course not. It does mean that if you really want to correct an issue you must fix the issue and then train as hard as you want. Just remember everything costs. My own personal dilemma when I stopped doing Olympic style weight lifting was "What now?" Adjustments were made and now training is not only better for me, its fun again.

I have learned to enjoy simply moving allowing myself from time to throw weights around. The difference is; I am not stiff after nor does my knee, back or foot hurt. I started to exercise my body properly by focusing on the Myofascial Meridians and it changed everything.

MYOFASCIAL MERIDIANS

Consisting of long lines throughout the body that make up our movement patterns used in both everyday, which is called foundational while in sport it is called adapted. The Myofascial meridians control both static and kinetic motor function. There is 10x more nerve receptors in the fascia then in muscle so its response is much higher than experts once thought. Posture is one of the main purposes of fascia along with holding our internal organs in place.

In this book we will primarily be focusing on the relation between the modern day hunter, gatherer and nurturer and the role fascia has on our health. We will be discussing in detail the different bodylines as we move thru the movements. There are 4 that we will focus on, these play key roles in the lives of our modern society. Once you learn and master them, you will see there role in all movements from swimming, running, even reaching for something off the shelf at home.

I am a man of few words and want to spend these pages getting to the exercises is the most important aspect. These movements will provide you with not just relief, release is attained which gives better movement and posture.

PREPPING'

This first section consists of movements done with bodyweight. It is designed to prepare the Myofascial bodylines. These movements should be done every morning, as they will help combat a day spent sitting. The sequence is one that I enjoy first thing in the morning before my partner or son is awake. My dogs have gotten used to it, but remember it is an adjustment for everyone in the house, so don't be surprised if your pets want to participate in the fun.

Take your time and learn one movement each day and by the end of the first week you will be able to put them together in a great sequence for waking the body and igniting the Lymphatic System.

OK. Here we go.

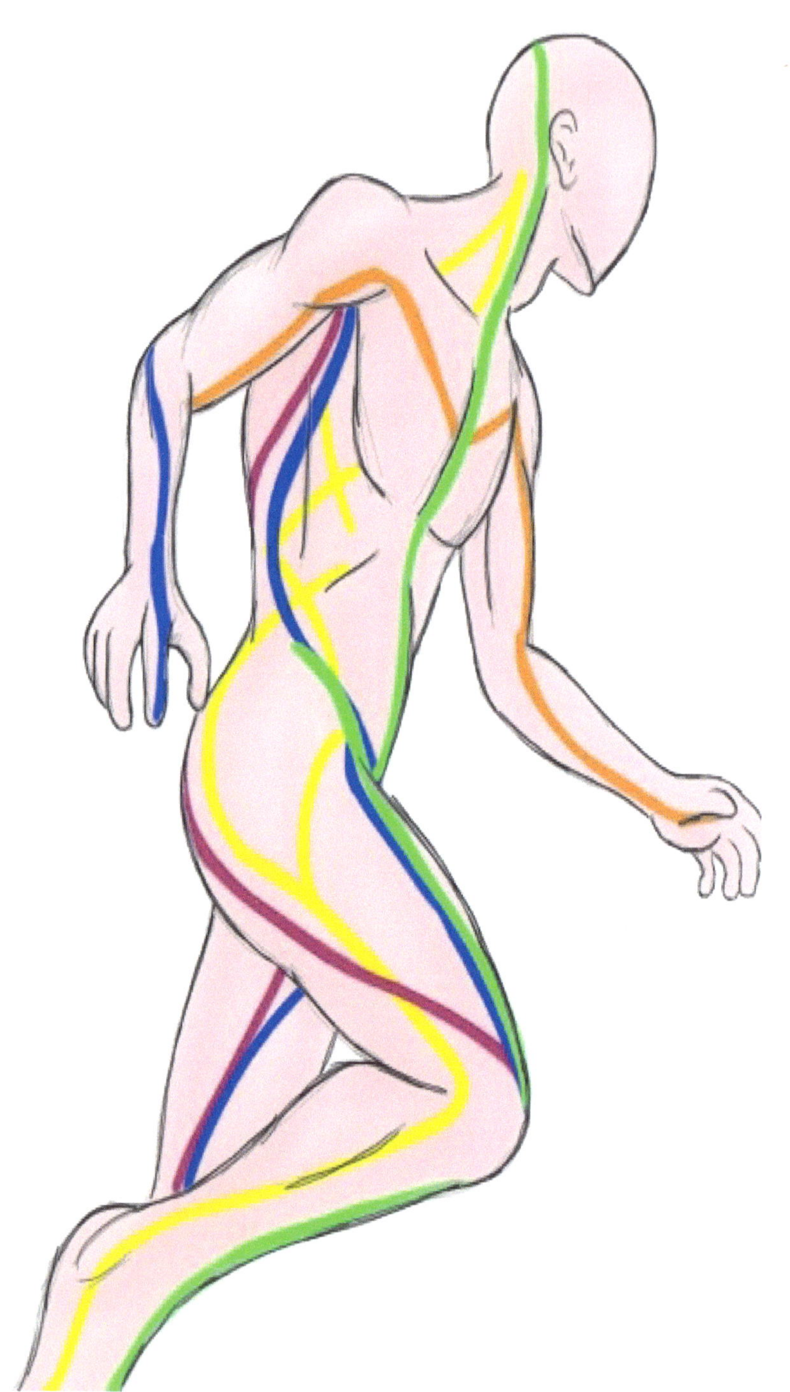

TRI-MOBILITY

A perfect way to warm up the Hips and also get your mind into the zone. Breathing is such a crucial piece to better mobility. Really focus on deep breathing using your diaphragm. Always remember to pin your sacrum to the floor.

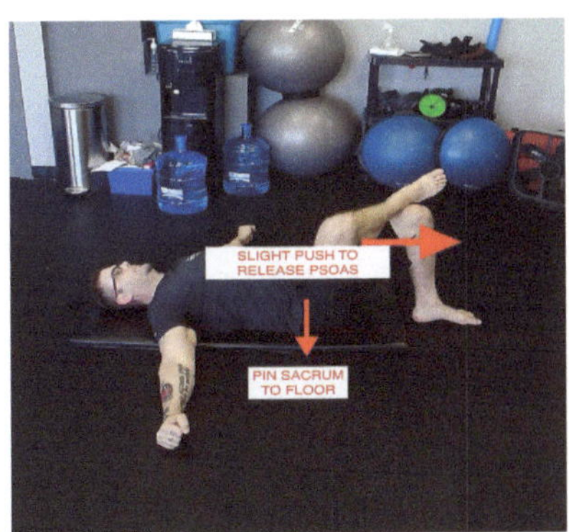

-Start by lying with knees bent. Feet directly under your knees, weight even from heel to toes. Bring one foot and rest it comfortably across the top of the opposite knee.

-Slowly pull the leg towards your chest, keeping pressure down. Try not to let your upper body lift; rather bring your lower body toward the torso. Range will depend on you
(Never force it)

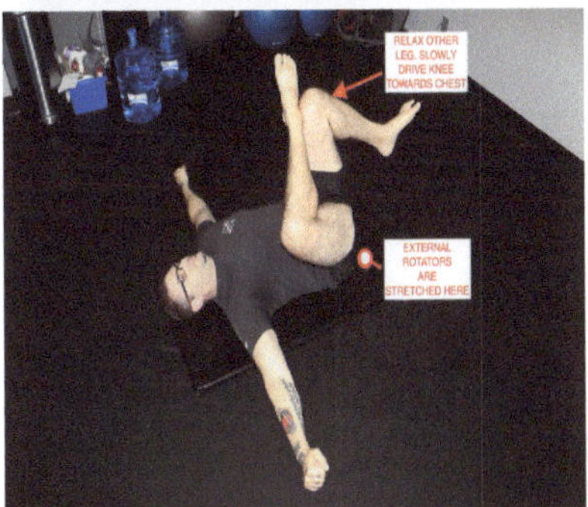

-Once back to neutral position (top pic) we are going to roll towards the leg that is planted. This requires tension in the thoracic.

-Press down into the ground with your fists and keep the pressure as you roll over till the foot lands flat (again do not force it)

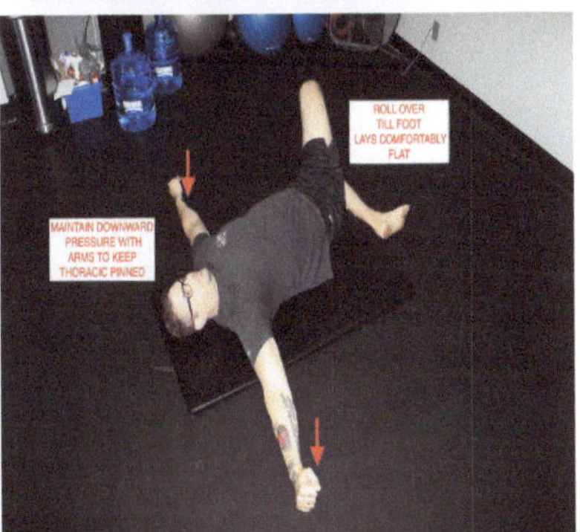

-Return once again to neutral position.

-The last movement is Glute Bridge. Posteriorly tilt pelvis to keep postural integrity.

-REPEAT SEQUENCE 5X each side

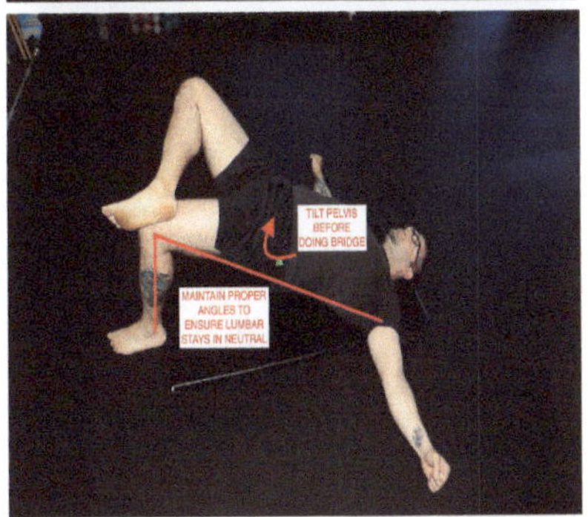

<u>90/90 hip openers</u>

For many people who sit behind a desk their hips get locked up at the Psoas and TFL due to constant shortening. The 90/90 is a great way to passively unlock these areas without aggressively stretching. The biggest thing with this is move with purpose; don't just let your leg flop down, move it there using the Adductor and Abductor bundles.

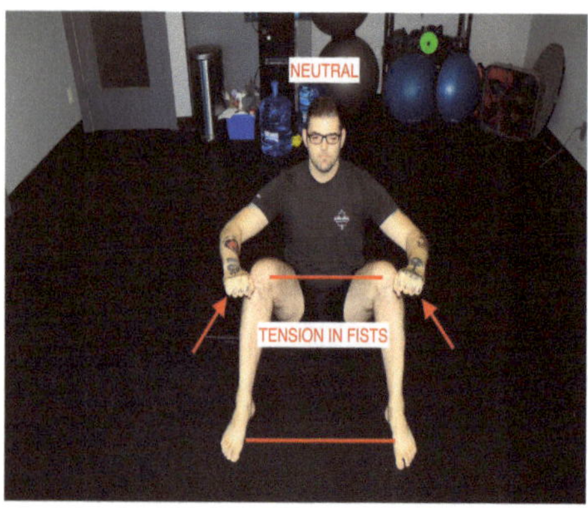

Start by getting comfortable. Because we are moving with purpose, we need to create some tension in areas we don't want moving. And in this case that's the Armline (think chest up)

While maintaining tension in Armline, slowly rotate your legs to the left, trying to touch the knees to the floor. Never force it. Just breath and move with purpose.

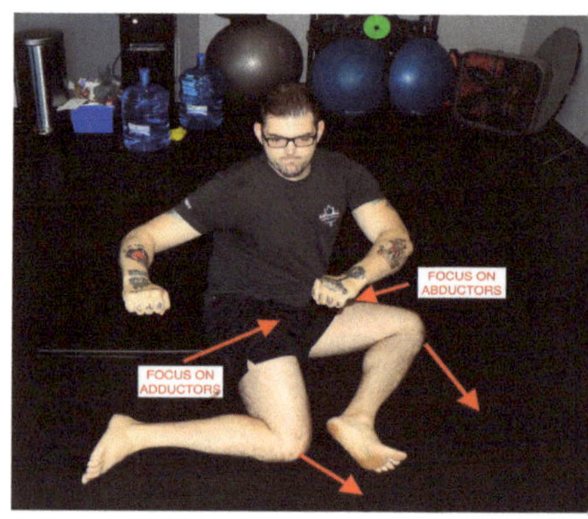

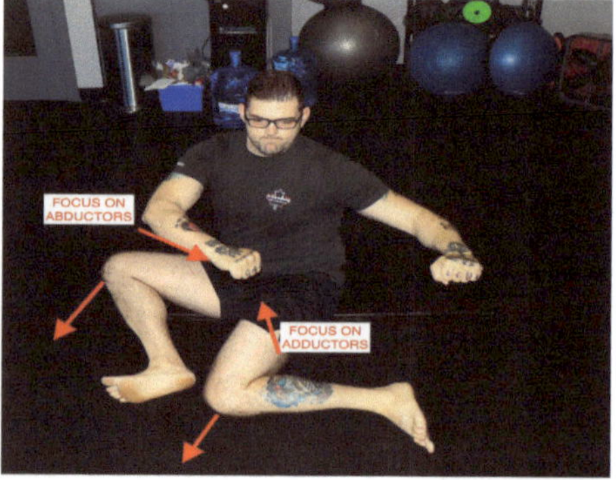

Return to neutral and rotate to the other side. Always maintaining tension in the Armline.

REPEAT 5X each side

CAT/COW in Quadruped position

One of my personal favourites. In the middle of a long day of writing this is my go to when I need a break.

-The most important position is the neutral.

-Ensure hands are directly under shoulders and Knees are directly under hips.

-Spine is in neutral line.

-Begin by taking a deep breathe in, expanding your diaphragm and as you let your breathe fall out lift the chest up by squeezing the shoulder blades together. (Don't drop your lumbar)

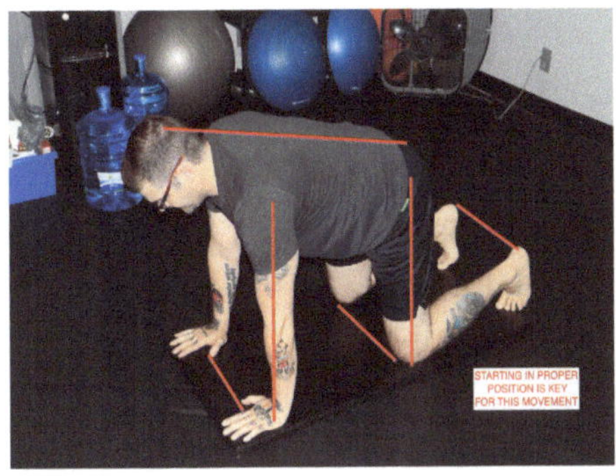

-Hold position until you begin to breath in again and begin to press your hands into the floor for leverage.

-Matching the out breathe press your thoracic to the ceiling and hollow out your abdomen (like vacuuming)

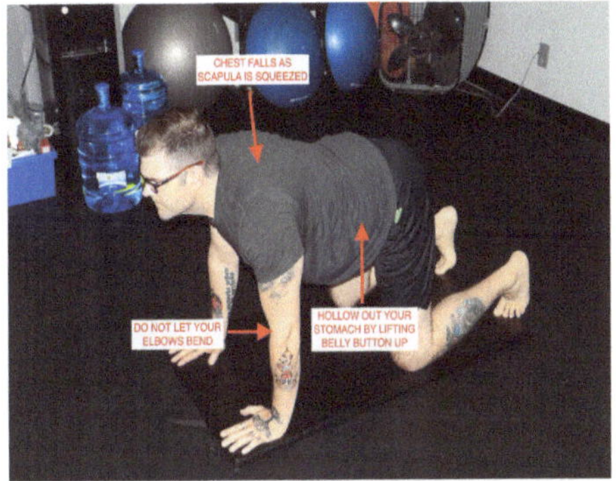

-When your thoracic is as expanded as it can get, posteriorly tilt your pelvis (as if you were tucking your tail)

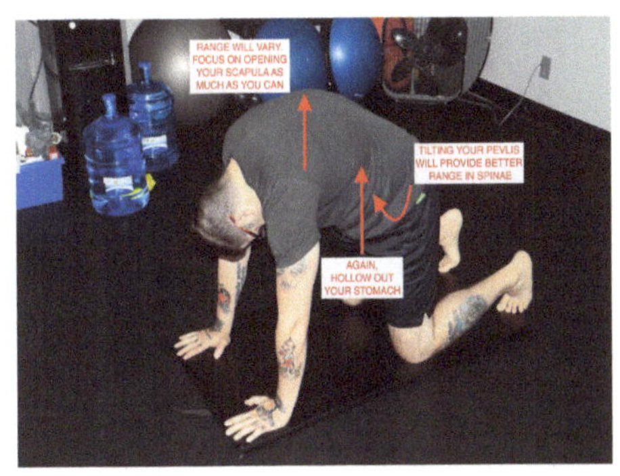

REPEAT THIS 5X and take your time.

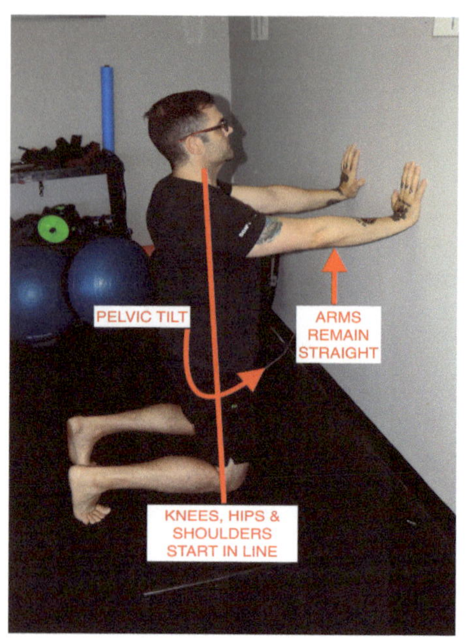

A great variation to the CAT/COW Quadruped is doing it on the wall. I like this version because it allows me to focus on hollowing my Abdomen.

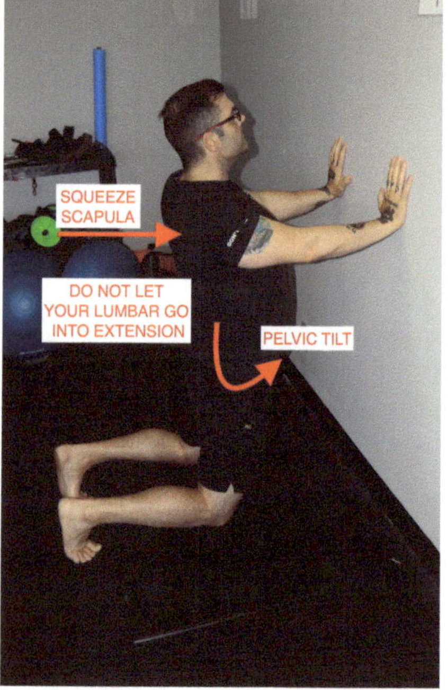

Most important aspect is to not allow your lumbar to go into hyperextension.

REPEAT 5X slowly

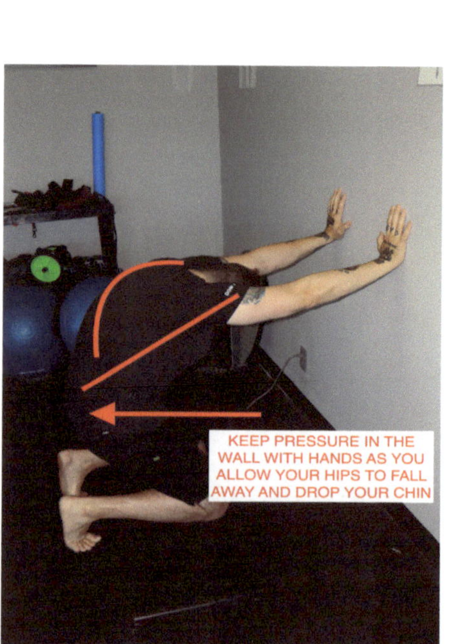

WALL LAT/PEC/SHOULDER

This Movement is such a great sequence to release those trigger points that tense up after sitting behind a desk all day. It is broken up into 2 pages so take your time and learn it well.

-Start by finding the distance from the wall.

-I do it by extending my arm straight out and where my fingers just touch is where I leave my feet.

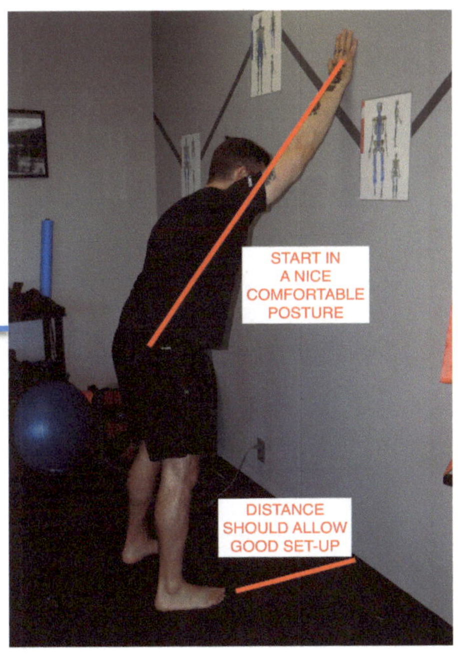

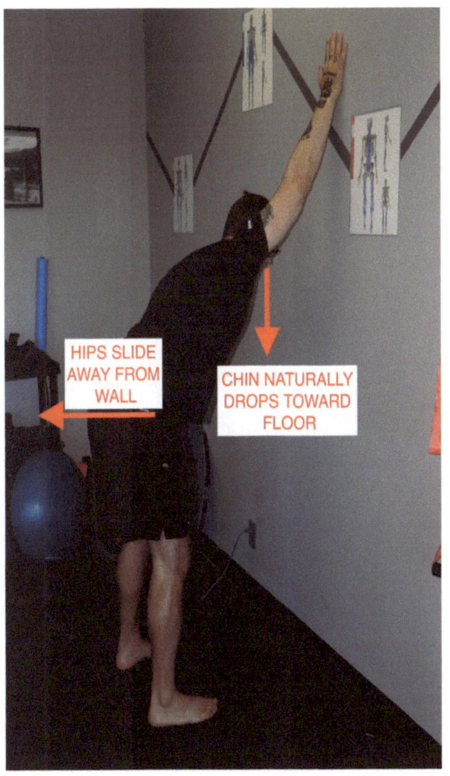

-First portion is to get the Pec Minor and Lat to open.

-Slowly let your hips slide back. Your hand should stay put. If it slides down the wall you have gone to far.

-Hold this position for a few seconds before moving to the next position.

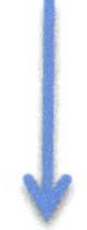

-Slowly crawl your opposite hand across the wall.

-Make sure to posteriorly tilt your pelvis first so you prevent lumbar rotation.

-The chest will turn with the hand and that is perfectly all right.

-Check in with your feet to double check the weight is even between heel and toes.

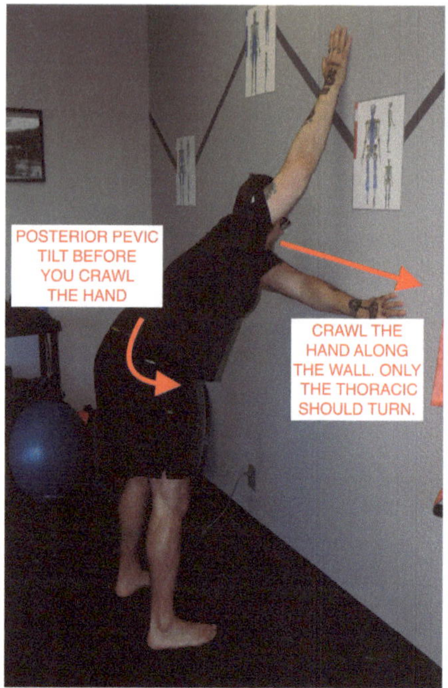

-Notice in the Back View the pull on the spiral line from the right hip across to the rear deltoid of the Left shoulder.

-Maintain posterior tilt for stability in Lumbar and Sacrum.

REPEAT 5X each side

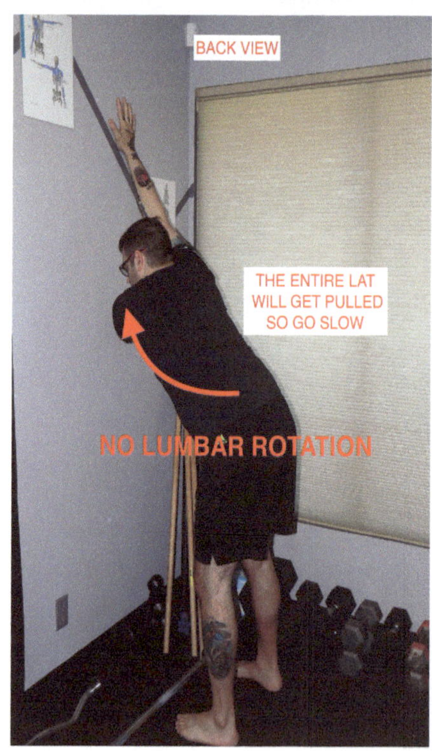

Developing proper connections when you are learning and mastering those PREPPING movements help you understand what is happening with your bodies balance. Pay attention to how your body feels, as you walk today and then in 2-3 weeks as you correct some dysfunction. The difference will be quite evident. It is really an amazing process as you begin to function better.

The PREPPING stage is designed for you to do daily. I personally do them in the morning as a way for me to get ready for the day. The movements are passive so you can do them multiple times throughout the day if you begin to feel stiff or find you are becoming more aware of postural positions, correct them right away. It takes time to optimize postural integrity as it took years of bad patterns to deform your body, it will take diligence and time to fix it.

In the next section we will explore some practical multi-line movements using Resistance. For the purpose of this book I have chosen to use Thera-band; It's easy to get and very convenient to travel with. There are a variety of tensions allowing you to constantly progress. I recommend movements beginning with the lightest tension in order to learn the patterns, becoming body aware of each movement, especially as it pertains to the Myofascial Bodylines. Let us take a closer look at the bodylines so you can get a better idea of what is what.

BODYLINES

<u>Superficial front and Superficial back lines</u>

These two lines play a role in every movement we do, whether foundational or adapted. The most important part is to understand that because your neck hurts, does not mean that is where the issue began. Rather, it can be a trigger 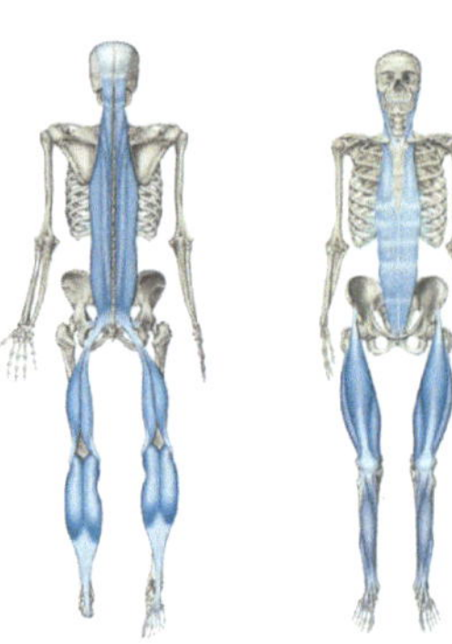 point to where the fascia has deformed enough to create tension and when fascia loses its elasticity it can make you extremely stiff. These lines also become confused and can switch primary roles due to prolonged sitting.

The superficial front line is under constant stress when sitting. The pec muscles, anterior delts, the forward flexion neck muscles, the abdominals, hip flexors and quad muscles are placed in a shortened position creating tension on the superficial back line to compensate and try to correct the postural vulnerability. When the body is in stagnation for long periods of time the fascia will adapt and deform in order to shape new patterns.

These two lines are an important piece to the healthy body pie. We must condition them accordingly. Lets first begin to release them so we can reshape our posture and start feeling great again.

The DEEP front line

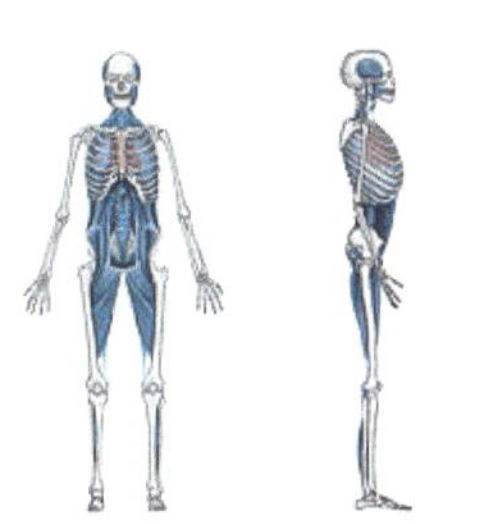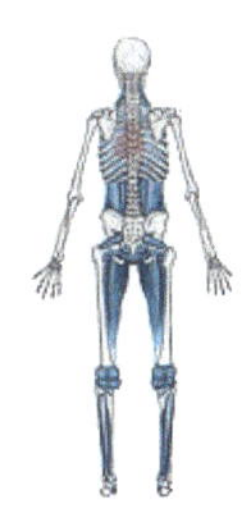

The Deep front line dictates our hip health. As you can see with the illustration the muscles of adduction are connected through a busy Myofascial freeway that controls forward movement, hip stability while in movement and of course the path in which our legs travel while walking or running. This line wreaks havoc on the lower back when we sit too long in forward bend I.E hunched over a computer.

When the Deep front line is not trained, it affects our breathing patterns. Our breaths become shallow, and taking in less oxygen, resulting in lowered brain function and poor circulation. Not to mention how important this line is for proper Lymphatic drainage.

The Lymphatic system, which is responsible for proper circulation and transporting healthy blood cells throughout the body, is dependant on movement to function properly and when it does not work right we are more susceptible to illness and fatigue. So though we are focusing on getting the body to feel and move better, the benefits reach beyond simple movements.

Now that we have PREPPED the body with some great body weight patterns lets add resistance to condition the fascia of the body and start reforming healthy postural integrity. The next section should be done one movement at a time. Do each one for a week until you have learned and mastered them all. Then you will be able to adjust and mix them into your weekly routine. Remember the PREPPING phase can be done daily I highly recommend this (you do them at the start of your day)

As with the PREPPING section, take your time and focus on the breathing. Stay aware of your Diaphragms expansion and contraction and mentally focus on how your body feels with each movement.

OK. Lets do this.

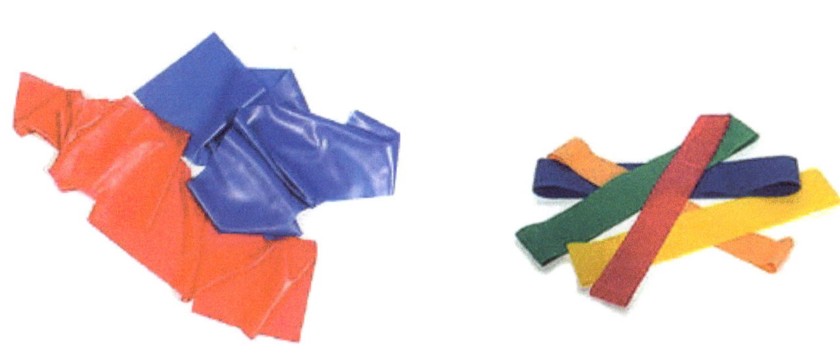

It is time to bring the bands out and get familiar with them. Included with the book (when purchased directly from NJLtraining) are a long light and medium band plus 1 looped band. Stick with the light band to begin with so you can really master the mechanics. Remember this is not about building strength; rather we are creating tension in certain areas while increasing mobility in other areas. It is planned this way and for best results we recommend following it.

<u>Bodyline activation drill</u>

This drill is one I go to before any resistance training, whether its bands or Kettlebells, I use this every time.

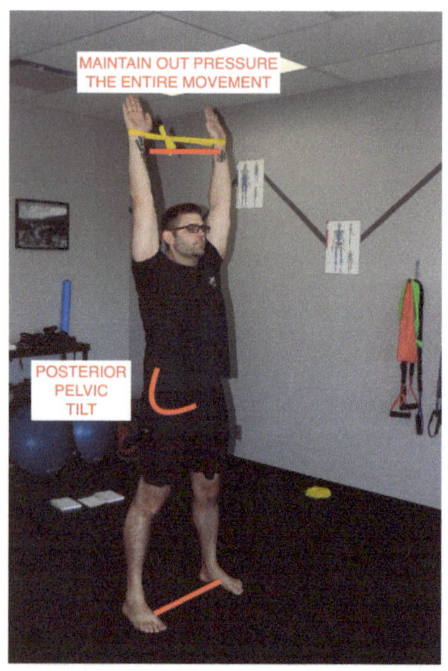

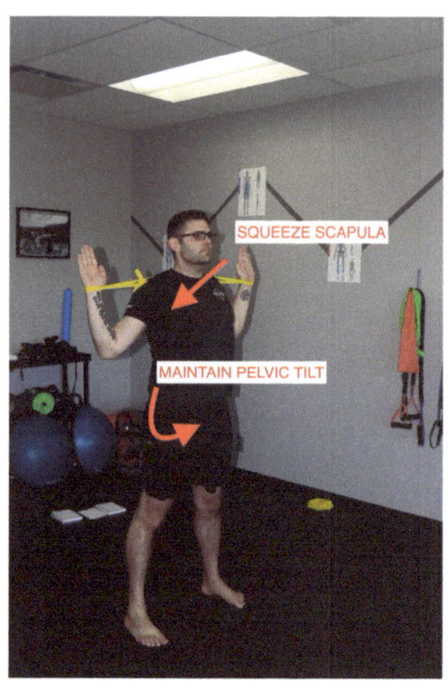

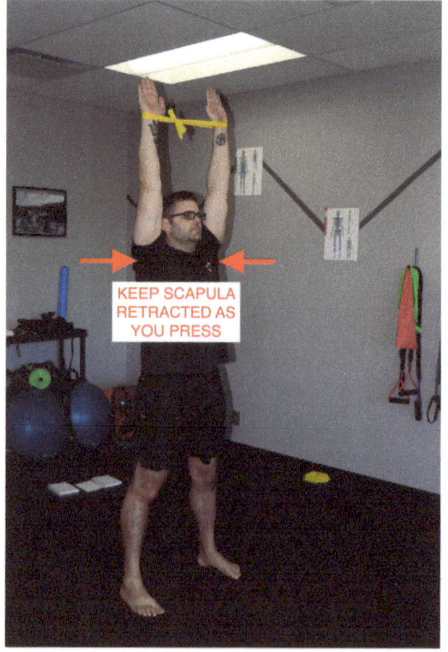

-The first part of the exercise is to lengthen the body while stabilizing the shoulder blades (Scapula).

-Start with arms extended overhead and create light outward pressure on the band.

-Slowly pull the elbows down to a W position, ensure you get full Scapula retraction.

-Complete by pressing hands back overhead.

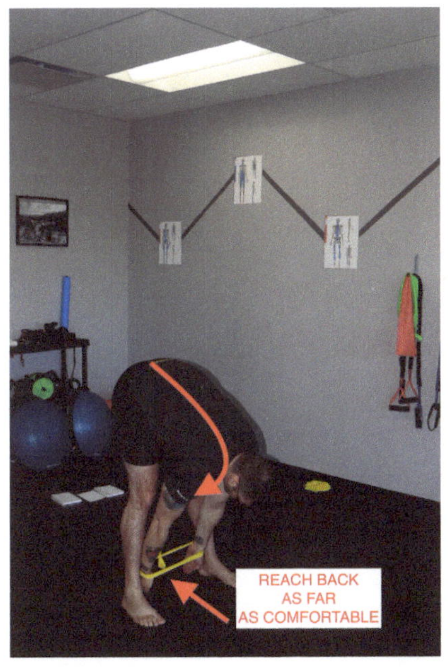

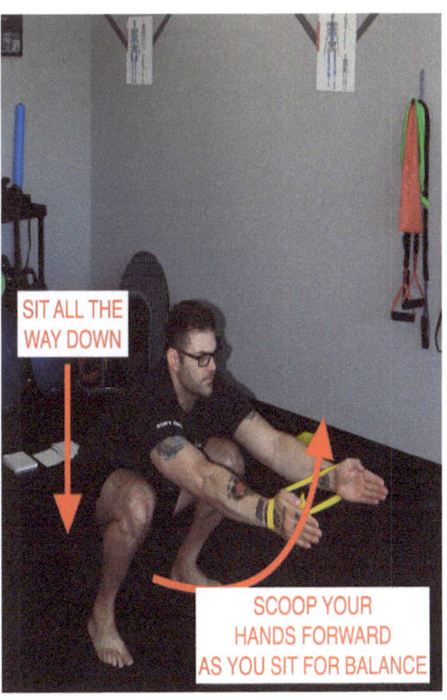

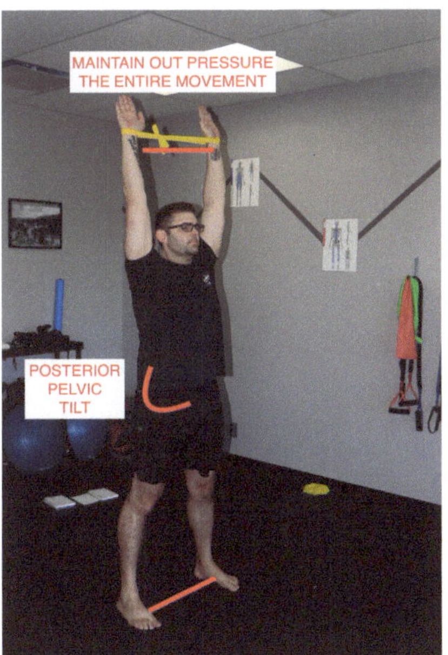

-Reach down and back between your legs; allow your back to round, as it is natural.

-As you sit your butt down to the floor scoop your hands forward and up (maintain outward tension on the band)

-To stand up, begin with your arms lifting and let your chest rise and then your hips and then your knees (avoid lifting your butt first)

REPEAT 5x

OH PULL/PRESS and SLIDE
Lets grab that long band and build some full body stability and increase core strength.

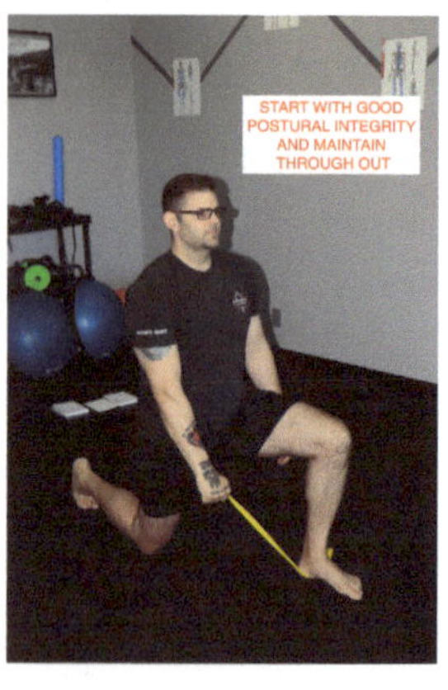

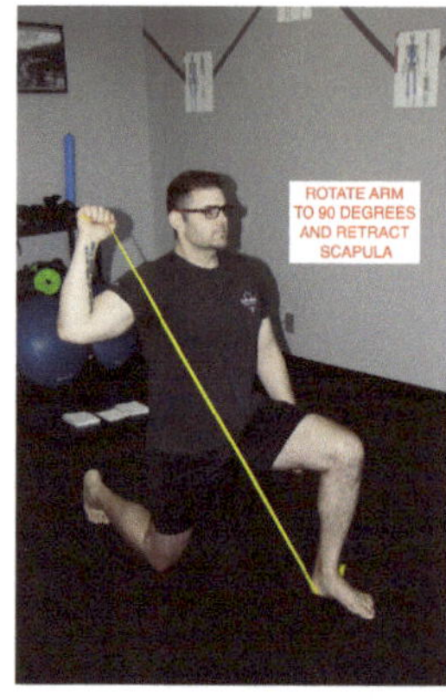

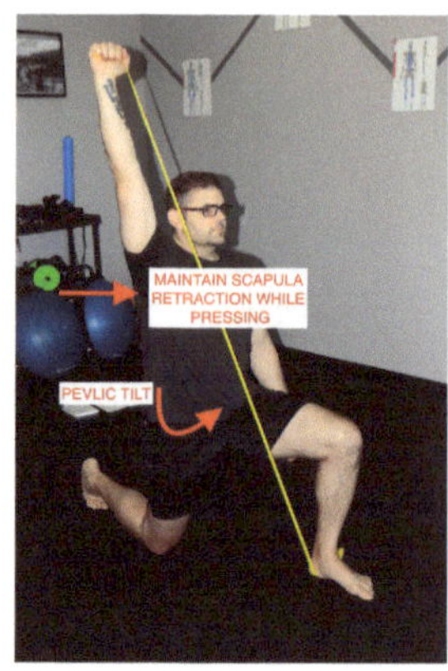

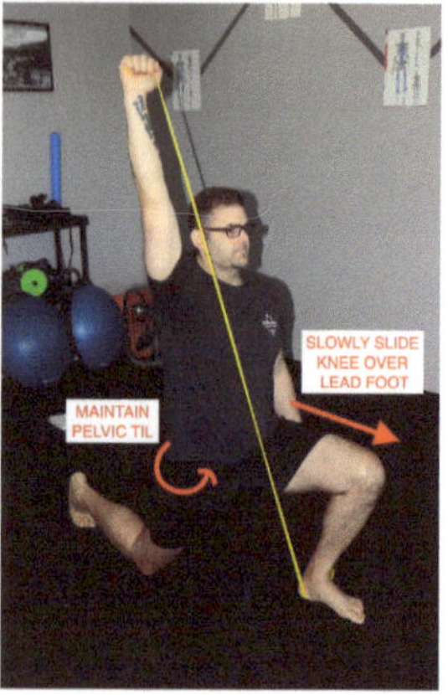

-Posture is everything here.

-Ensure head, shoulders, hips and knees are in a vertical line.

-Pull elbow back to parallel and rotate forearm to a vertical.

-Posteriorly tilt pelvis and press hand overhead slowly, focusing on maintaining Scapula retraction.

-Keeping posterior tilt, slide entire torso forward till front knee is over or past foot (if tilt is not maintained, reset and only slide till it is)

REPEAT 5X each side

<h1 style="text-align:center"><u>ALTERNATING butterfly</u></h1>

For many people back problems are a result of poor GLUTE MED stability and function. This exercise is great after a long day when the lower back feels stiff.

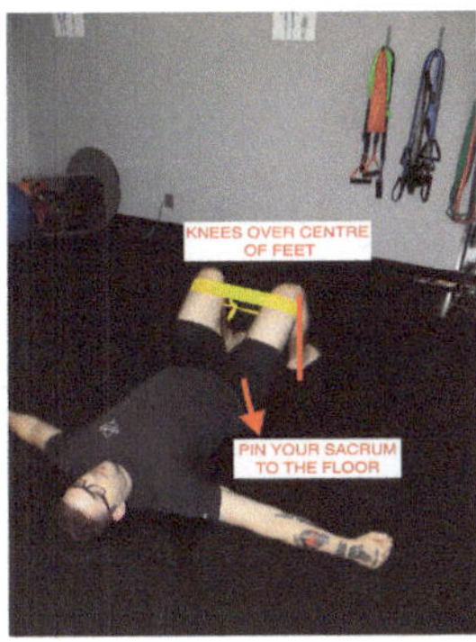

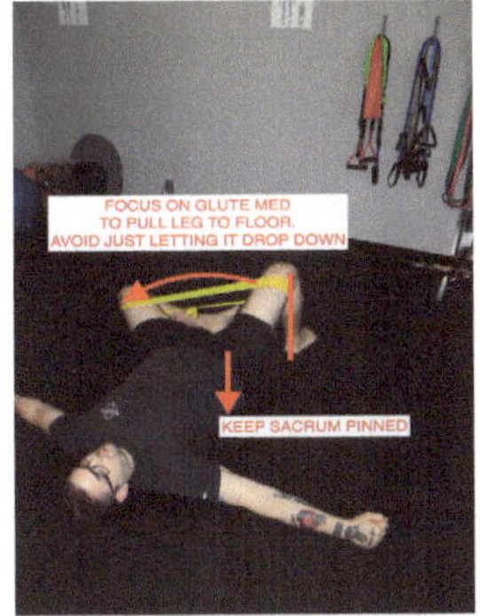

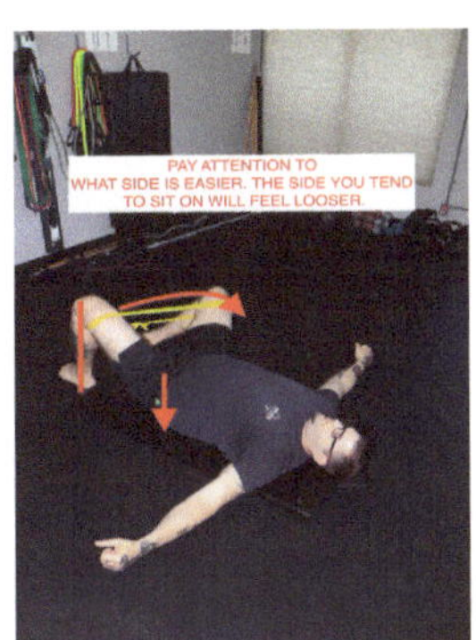

This sequence is really nice to end the day. After I have been standing all day and my back feels stiff I like to do this for about ten minutes. You don't need that much time if you don't have it, I just enjoy doing it really slowly and taking about 2-3 full breaths each rep.

-The first position must be comfortable. Knees above the heels, pelvis posteriorly tilted and sacrum pinned.

-Before you slowly abduct your leg ensure you drive your fists into the floor to brace your thoracic and minimize any shifting of weight.

-Return to start position and readjust if needed and repeat on other side

REPEAT at least 5x each side

Congratulations you have completed the book. I hope you have made the movements a part of your daily life and I know that if you have, your body has begun to feel much better. It is important to remember this book is not intended to be a strenuous workout; rather I want to help you release the tension that is built up from hours upon hours spent behind a desk.

As I mentioned before, take your time with these movements, really learn and master them so that when you go to the gym, enjoy a hike, or any other activity; you can do it pain free. Life is movement. It is time to treat your body the way it was designed. You can live a quality life by learning to move more efficiently.

Thank you so much for taking the time to read this book.

*A special thanks to David Lewry Photography for the great pics.
A huge thanks to my beautiful partner for always being supportive, I get do what I love because of you. And to my family, I can never thank you enough.

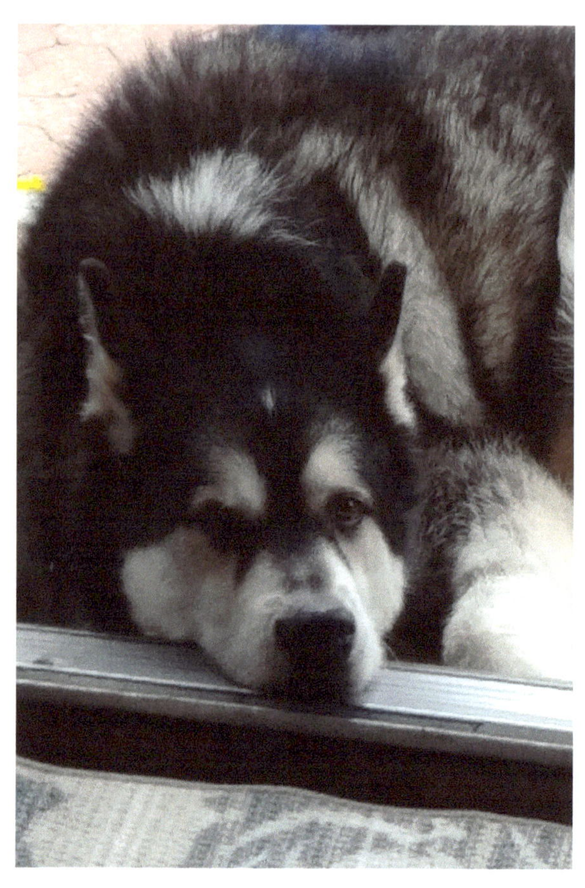

WRITTEN BY:
NJLtraining
Active Myofascial Decompression Therapy

Photos done by:
David Lewry Photography